Drugs and Sports

Locating the Author's Main Idea

Drugs and Sports

Locating the Author's Main Idea

Curriculum Consultant: JoAnne Buggey, Ph.D.
College of Education, University of Minnesota

By Carol O'Sullivan

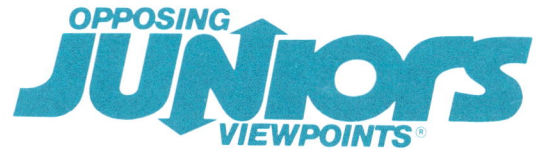

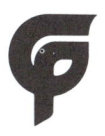

Greenhaven Press, Inc.
Post Office Box 289009
San Diego, CA 92128-9009

Titles in the opposing viewpoints juniors series:

Smoking   Death Penalty
Gun Control   Drugs and Sports
Animal Rights   Toxic Wastes
AIDS   Patriotism
Alcohol   Working Mothers
Immigration   Poverty

Cover photos: J. Myers/H. Armstrong Roberts, Camerique

Library of Congress Cataloging-in-Publication Data

O'Sullivan, Carol, 1945-
  Drugs and sports : locating the author's main idea / by Carol
O'Sullivan : curriculum consultant, JoAnne Buggey.
    p.   cm. — (Opposing viewpoints juniors)
  Summary: Presents opposing viewpoints on the issues surrounding
the use of drugs by athletes, steroid abuse, and drug testing.
Includes critical thinking skill activities
  ISBN 0-89908-495-8
  1. Doping in sports—Juvenile literature. 2. Athletes—Drug use—
Juvenile literature. 3. Critical thinking—Juvenile literature.
[1. Athletes—Drug use. 2. Drug abuse. 3. Critical thinking.]
  I. Title. II. Series.
RC1230.078   1989
362.29'08'8796—dc20   89-36322
                                                           CIP
                                                            AC

No part of this book may be reproduced or used in any other form
or by any other means, electrical, mechanical or otherwise, including,
but not limited to photocopy, recording or any information storage and
retrieval system, without prior written permission from the publisher.

Copyright 1989 by Greenhaven Press, Inc.

CONTENTS

The Purpose of This Book: **An Introduction to Opposing Viewpoints**............................6
Skill Introduction: **Locating the Author's Main Idea**............................7
Sample Viewpoint A: **I think drugs should be allowed in sports**............................8
Sample Viewpoint B: **I think drugs should be banned in sports**............................9
Analyzing the
Sample Viewpoints: **Locating the Author's Main Idea**............................10

Chapter 1

Preface: Can Steroids Be Used Safely?............................11
Viewpoint 1: **Steroids can be used safely**............................12
    paraphrased views of *Ron Hale*
Viewpoint 2: **Steroids cannot be used safely**............................14
    paraphrased views of the *American College of Sports Medicine*
Critical Thinking Skill 1: **Locating the Author's Main Idea**............................16

Chapter 2

Preface: Should Drugs Be Allowed in Sports?............................17
Viewpoint 3: **Drugs should be allowed in sports**............................18
    paraphrased views of *Norman Fost*
Viewpoint 4: **Drugs should not be allowed in sports**............................22
    paraphrased views of *Thomas H. Murray*
Critical Thinking Skill 2: **Identifying the Main Idea in Editorial Cartoons**............................26

Chapter 3

Preface: Should Athletes Be Tested for Drug Use?............................27
Viewpoint 5: **Athletes should be tested for drugs**............................28
    paraphrased views of *Robert Voy*
Viewpoint 6: **Athletes should not be tested for drugs**............................30
    paraphrased views of *Bryan Burwell*
Critical Thinking Skill 3: **Developing the Main Idea**............................32

THE PURPOSE OF THIS BOOK

An Introduction to Opposing Viewpoints

When people disagree, it is hard to figure out who is right. You may decide one person is right just because the person is your friend or relative. But this is not a very good reason to agree or disagree with someone. It is better if you try to understand why these people disagree. On what main points do they differ? Read or listen to each person's argument carefully. Separate the facts and opinions that each person presents. Finally, decide which argument best matches what you think. This process, examining an argument without emotion, is part of what critical thinking is all about.

This is not easy. Many things make it hard to understand and form opinions. People's values, ages, and experiences all influence the way they think. This is why learning to read and think critically is an invaluable skill. Opposing Viewpoints Juniors books will help you learn and practice skills to improve your ability to read critically. By reading opposing views on an issue, you will become familiar with methods people use to attempt to convince you that their point of view is right. And you will learn to separate the authors' opinions from the facts they present.

Each Opposing Viewpoints Juniors book focuses on one critical thinking skill that will help you judge the views presented. Some of these skills are telling fact from opinion, recognizing propaganda techniques, and locating and analyzing the main idea. These skills will allow you to examine opposing viewpoints more easily.

Each viewpoint in this book is paraphrased from the original to make it easier to read. The viewpoints are placed in a running debate and are always placed with the pro view first.

SKILL INTRODUCTION

Locating the Author's Main Idea

Authors include many ideas in their writing. But each sentence, each paragraph, and even each book they write should contain one main idea. For example, the main idea of this book is that the use of drugs in sports is a much-debated issue.

Locating the author's main idea, whether it is within the sentence, paragraph, or entire piece of writing, is a basic reading skill. It is important because it allows readers to identify the theme of an author's writing. It also allows readers to understand the main point an author is trying to make about the theme.

In this Opposing Viewpoints Juniors book, you will be asked to analyze specific paragraphs to locate the main idea. Sometimes the main idea is placed at the beginning of the paragraph. Sometimes it is placed somewhere within the paragraph, or even at the end. For example:

> People have destroyed the homes of many animals by cutting down trees in the rain forest to use for construction. They have also cut short the food supply of many grass-eating animals by using prairie land for building homes and businesses. People's use of the land is threatening the existence of many animals.

The main idea of this paragraph is placed at the end. It is that people's use of the land is threatening the existence of many animals.

When you begin reading the paragraph, you might think the first sentence is the main idea. If it is, then the other sentences in the paragraph will support it in some way. They might explain the idea more specifically or give examples or reasons.

Read sentence two. Does it do any of these things? No. In fact, sentence two is very much like sentence one. Sentence two even says *also,* which suggests that the two sentences are giving two ideas about the same topic.

Now read the last sentence. It is a general statement about the topic of destroying animals' habitats, while the first two are specific examples of this. The last sentence in this paragraph is the topic sentence. The other two sentences support this last sentence.

If you outlined this paragraph, it would look like this:

1. People's use of the land is threatening the existence of many animals.

    A. (Example 1) People have destroyed the homes of many animals by cutting down trees in the rain forest to use for construction.

    B. (Example 2) They have also cut short the food supply of many grass-eating animals by using prairie land for building homes and businesses.

Most paragraphs can be outlined in this way. By reading a paragraph carefully, you should be able to tell which sentence presents the main idea and which sentences explain or support it in some way. Outlining the paragraph may help you figure this out.

We asked two students to write one paragraph each in which they state their main ideas about drug use by athletes. Examine the following viewpoints to locate the main ideas.

SAMPLE VIEWPOINT A *Christy*

I think drugs should be allowed in sports.

All people, including athletes, have the right to do anything they want with their own bodies. After all, America is a free country. People can even do things that might hurt them. This means people should be able to take drugs, as long as the drugs aren't illegal.

SAMPLE VIEWPOINT B *Steve*

I think drugs should be banned in sports.

It's not fair when some athletes take drugs to make them run faster or lift more weight and other athletes don't. Athletes who don't take the drugs can't win against those who do. All the practicing in the world isn't going to help them compete against someone who takes drugs. Athletes shouldn't be allowed to take drugs.

ANALYZING THE SAMPLE VIEWPOINTS

Christy and Steve have very different opinions about drug use in sports. Each presents one main idea in his or her viewpoint.

Christy:
MAIN IDEA

All people, including athletes, have the right to do anything they want with their own bodies.

Steve:
MAIN IDEA

Athletes shouldn't be allowed to take drugs.

Christy's main idea comes at the beginning of her statement, while Steve's main idea comes at the end.

As you continue to read through the viewpoints in this book, remember to look for the main idea of the specified paragraphs.

CHAPTER 1

PREFACE: Can Steroids Be Used Safely?

Steroids are powerful artificial or natural chemicals that are related to male hormones. A hormone is a product of living cells that affects other body cells in some way. Some hormones, for example, promote growth.

Steroids can be used to treat medical problems. They help heal injuries to the body's tissues, they help correct bone disorders, and they help cure certain diseases.

Steroids have another use that is not related to medicine. They are used as performance-enhancing drugs. A performance-enhancing drug can help an athlete perform better at his or her sport. These drugs can make athletes stronger and faster than athletes who do not take the drugs. Many athletes use steroids because they believe steroids increase their muscle size and thus make them stronger than their opponents. This advantage, they believe, helps them to win.

Many people argue that athletes should not be allowed to use steroids. These people say that steroids are dangerous and that they should be used only to treat illnesses. Opponents of steroid use point out the dangers steroids pose to an athlete's health. Liver and heart diseases can result from steroid use. Also, men can develop female breasts, and women can develop facial hair from using steroids. Finally, people who use steroids sometimes suffer from extreme moodiness and violent behavior.

Other people argue that taking steroids in small doses is not dangerous to a person's health. These people add that even if steroids were dangerous, athletes should have the freedom to do whatever they want with their own bodies.

When reading the following viewpoints, locate the author's main idea in the specified paragraphs.

VIEWPOINT 1 Steroids can be used safely

Editor's Note: This viewpoint is paraphrased from an article by Ron Hale, a former U.S. weight-lifting champion. In this viewpoint, Mr. Hale discusses why he thinks athletes should be allowed to use steroids.

The main idea in this paragraph is stated in the first sentence.

The main idea in this paragraph is stated near the end of the paragraph. It is that athletes are pressured into taking steroids.

Steroids are perfectly safe when taken in small doses. I have been taking them for twenty years. I have undergone every possible medical test. These tests have shown that steroids have not hurt me in any way.

Communist countries give steroids to their athletes. If American athletes did not take them, they would not be able to perform as well as the communist athletes. Even if steroids were not safe, athletes would be pressured to take them anyway. They need steroids to compete with other athletes who are taking them.

I know steroids help an athlete to perform better. I started taking steroids because I thought my performance was slowing. I was 5 feet five inches tall and weighed 155 pounds. I could lift a total of 1,150 pounds. Three years later, after using steroids, I weighed 165 pounds, and I won the U.S. senior power-lifting title by lifting 1,425 pounds. In all, I have won nine state titles. I think I would have won most of them without steroids. But there is no way I could have won the national title without them.

I have been off steroids for nine months. But when I return to lifting, I will use them again, especially if other weight-lifters are using them.

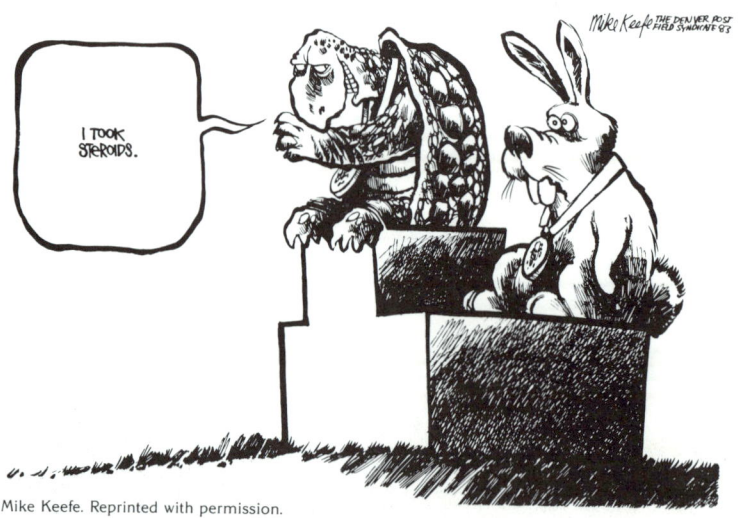

Mike Keefe. Reprinted with permission.

12 JUNIORS

People have the right to do whatever they want with their own bodies. No one, including sports organizations, should tell us we cannot take steroids.

Brian Bosworth, a football linebacker, was suspended by the National Collegiate Athletic Association (NCAA) for taking steroids. Bosworth's suspension was unfair. He was taking steroids for an injury. But even if he were not taking them for an injury, it was his constitutional right to take steroids. After all, steroids do not alter the mind in any way. Taking them is not habit-forming.

If Bosworth feels steroids help his performance, that is his business. The NCAA should stop worrying about athletes who take steroids. They should concentrate on athletes who take other drugs, such as marijuana.

Steroids can be used safely and with good results by adults. But teenagers should never use them. Steroids stunt growth and cause other damage to young people. I would not let my 12-year-old son take them. But if he comes to me ten years from now when he is fully grown and asks if he should take them, I will say yes. As long as he does it under a doctor's care, he will have no problems.

Steroids can be used safely. Just be smart about it.

Which sentence best expresses the author's main idea in this paragraph?

What is the author's main idea in this paragraph?

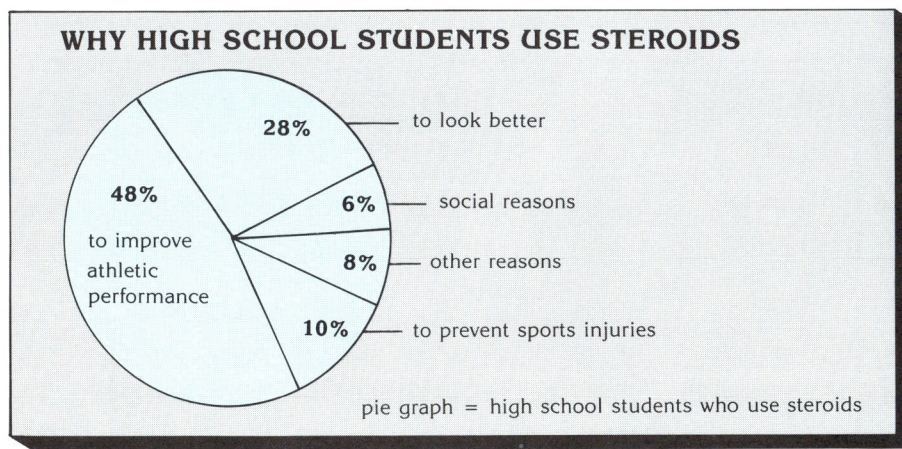

Are people free to hurt themselves?

Do you agree with the author that people should have the right to do whatever they want with their own bodies? Do you agree that people have this right even if what they want to do might hurt them? Why or why not?

VIEWPOINT 2 Steroids cannot be used safely

> **Editor's Note:** This viewpoint is paraphrased from an article by the American College of Sports Medicine. In it, the authors argue that steroids are dangerous and should not be used.

The authors' main idea in this paragraph may be a little more difficult to locate. Read the paragraph carefully and decide which sentence best expresses it.

Steroids may have some positive effects on the body. Test results show that low doses of steroids taken during weight training increase strength and muscle mass. But these increases are also affected by other things besides steroids. Diet, amount of physical training, and a person's outlook on life all contribute to successful weight training.

Perhaps steroids do affect the body in some positive ways. But the problems caused by these drugs outweigh the benefits. One problem caused by steroids is liver damage.

The liver plays a role in breaking down many drugs so that the body can use them. A high intake of steroids can overload the liver and result in liver failure. In fact, studies using animals and humans have proved that taking too many steroids can severely damage the liver.

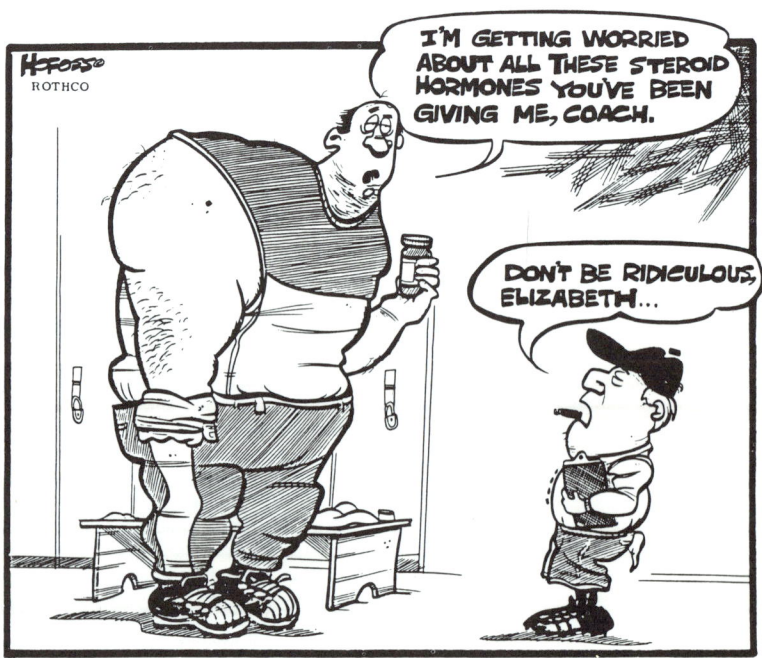
© Hofoss/Rothco

14 JUNIORS

Steroids can also cause liver diseases. Peliosis hepatitis—the development of blood-filled cysts that can burst and lead to liver failure—is associated with steroid use. Jaundice—bile in the blood causing yellowing of the skin and eyeballs—is also linked with steroids. Finally, liver tumors have been found in some patients who have taken steroids. Most of these tumors were non-cancerous. However, cancerous liver tumors have been found in at least one young male bodybuilder.

Locate the authors' main idea in this paragraph.

Besides causing liver problems, steroids can also lead to heart disease and other heart problems. Animal research has shown that steroid use can lead to damage of the heart muscle itself.

Men who take steroids sometimes develop large breasts. Females also experience problems with steroid use. Some women have reported thinning hair, deepening of the voice, reduced breast size, and even growth of facial hair. The use of steroids affects the physical appearance of both men and women.

What is the authors' main idea in this paragraph?

Other undesirable physical effects associated with steroid use include mental as well as physical problems. Some people become depressed. Others become moody and hostile.

Which sentence best expresses the authors' main idea in this paragraph?

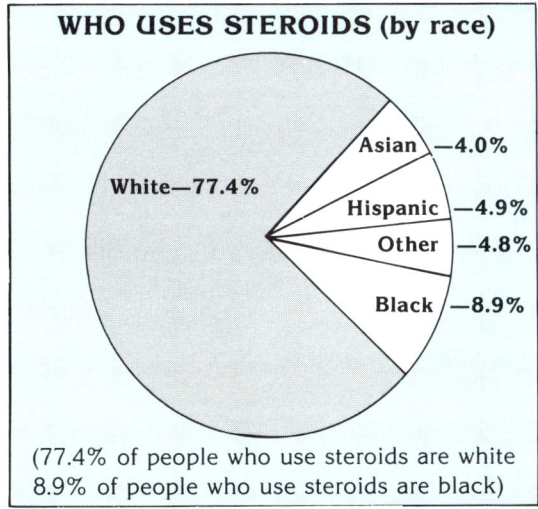

WHO USES STEROIDS (by race)
White—77.4%
Asian—4.0%
Hispanic—4.9%
Other—4.8%
Black—8.9%

(77.4% of people who use steroids are white
8.9% of people who use steroids are black)

SOURCE: JAMA, Dec. 1988

Are steroids safe?

After reading these two viewpoints, do you think steroid use is safe or unsafe? Why? Which viewpoint did you find most convincing? Why?

DRUGS AND SPORTS **15**

CRITICAL THINKING SKILL 1

Locating the Author's Main Idea

The following paragraphs each contain one main idea. Below each paragraph are three sentences, one of which best expresses the main idea of the paragraph. Circle the sentence that best expresses the main idea.

EXAMPLE: Many athletes use drugs. Some use alcohol to relax them after a game. Others use cocaine and marijuana to escape the pressures of competing. Still others use performance-enhancing drugs such as steroids to help them become better athletes.

    a. Athletes are drug addicts.
    b. Many athletes use drugs.
    c. Athletes smoke marijuana.

The answer is b. The author's main idea is that many athletes use drugs.

1. Steroids have been linked to liver tumors, kidney and liver problems, hostile behavior, and inability to have children. Also, recent studies have linked steroid use to depression. The father of a teenager who committed suicide says that his son's bouts with depression began when he started taking steroids. Steroids can have harmful effects on the body.

    a. Steroids can have harmful effects on the body.
    b. Steroids cause cancer.
    c. Steroid use causes teenagers to commit suicide.

2. Ben Johnson, an Olympic sprinter, was disqualified from the 1988 Olympics. He was stripped of his medals for using drugs. But Johnson's disqualification was unfair. Twenty other athletes tested positive for steroids, and they were not disqualified. The reason given was that these other athletes were not taking enough of the steroids to cause the Olympic Committee to suspend them.

    a. Ben Johnson is an Olympic sprinter.
    b. Ben Johnson's disqualification from the Olympics was unfair.
    c. Twenty athletes tested positive for steroids at the 1988 Olympics.

CHAPTER 2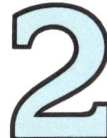

PREFACE: Should Drugs Be Allowed in Sports?

Most people agree that performance-enhancing drugs help athletes perform better. These drugs, including steroids, caffeine, and even some drugs used to treat diseases, can make athletes stronger.

But many people believe the use of any performance-enhancing drugs should be forbidden. They argue that athletes who take these drugs have an advantage over athletes who do not take them. Athletes, they say, sometimes win because they are taking drugs rather than because they are the best at their sports.

Other people think drugs should be allowed in sports. These people do not accept the argument that drugs should be forbidden because they give some athletes an advantage. After all, they say, many athletes already have natural advantages over other athletes. Some athletes are stronger, taller, and faster than others. According to people who support drug use in sports, forbidding drugs because they cause inequality among athletes does not make sense. Athletes are already unequal.

The following viewpoints debate the use of drugs in sports.

VIEWPOINT 3 Drugs should be allowed in sports

Editor's Note: This viewpoint is paraphrased from an article by Norman Fost, director of the Program in Medical Ethics at the University of Wisconsin. Dr. Fost personally opposes the use of drugs in sports; however, he believes the reasons for banning drugs from sports are poor ones.

Which sentence best states the author's main idea in this paragraph? Do the remaining sentences in the paragraph support the main idea? Why or why not?

Many people believe that performance-enhancing drugs, including steroids, should be banned from sports. They argue that these drugs give athletes unfair advantage over athletes who do not use drugs. But there is a problem with this argument. Inequality among athletes is not necessarily unfair.

We do not think it is unfair that Kareem Abdul-Jabbar is taller than most other basketball players. Nor do we consider it unfair that Martina Navratilova is stronger and faster than other tennis players. Some athletes are just born with bodies that are naturally stronger, faster, or taller than most. But we do not keep athletes with these natural advantages from competing with athletes who do not have these advantages.

WHEN DO COLLEGE ATHLETES BEGIN USING DRUGS?

	During Junior High Or Before	During High School	During First-Year College	During Later College Years
Cigarettes*	41	34	14	12
Smokeless	16	53	24	7
Alcohol	24	65	8	3
Marijuana/hashish*	25	58	10	6
Cocaine	4	42	24	30
Psychedelics*	13	44	21	20
Barbiturates/Tranquilizers*	31	31	17	17
Amphetamines*	8	58	21	14

*Percentages do not total 100% because of rounding.

SOURCE: Delaware Medical Journal

18 JUNIORS

Even when the advantage is a result of human decision rather than natural qualities, we do not consider it unfair. Much of Abdul-Jabbar's advantage is that he practices long hours. We do not consider this unfair to other players who choose not to practice so long.

It is true that in some sports opponents have to be fairly matched. Boxers and wrestlers do not compete against bigger or stronger opponents. Women are not usually matched against men. But most sports allow unevenly matched opponents to compete against each other.

Athletes also eat special food as well as take certain drugs to enhance their performance. Athletes follow special diets, drink special fluids, and take vitamins and minerals to make them healthier and better able to compete. Why not ban these substances from sports? Certainly a healthful diet and extra vitamins will give an athlete an advantage over an athlete who eats nothing but junk food. Yet, no one considers it unfair that athletes try to gain an advantage by improving their health.

> **Which sentence best expresses the author's main idea in this paragraph?**

People who oppose the use of drugs in sports argue that drugs are harmful to athletes. But this is not a good argument, either. In many sports, the risk of competing is greater than the risk of taking certain banned drugs. For example, many football players suffer permanent injuries while playing football. Yet, we are not worried about the health of athletes who participate in dangerous sports.

> **Consider the ideas carefully in this paragraph. Which idea best expresses the main point the author is trying to make?**

The truth is that the American public enjoys sports that involve high risk. It tolerates death and disability because Americans believe in personal freedom. They believe people have the right to do whatever they want with their own bodies. That includes participating in a dangerous sport, competing against a bigger, stronger opponent, or taking a performance-enhancing drug.

Which sentences support the main idea that athletes do not have to take drugs?

What is the author's main idea in this paragraph?

A final argument people use to oppose the use of drugs in sports is that athletes are not really free to choose to take drugs or not. They are supposedly forced into taking drugs because they cannot compete without drugs.

But athletes do not have to take drugs. They will not lose anything they already own—such as their health, or property, or basic rights—because they do not take them. The most they will lose is a gold medal or money. But these are not things they already own.

Athletes will lose nothing if they refuse to take performance-enhancing drugs, but they gain something if they do take these drugs. They gain an opportunity to improve themselves. Admittedly, there are health risks, but opportunities are usually accompanied by risks.

Perhaps the answer to making sure athletes are more fairly matched is to offer the same advantages, including performance-enhancing drugs, to all athletes. An example of this happened in pole-vaulting. Athletes found that fiberglass poles helped them

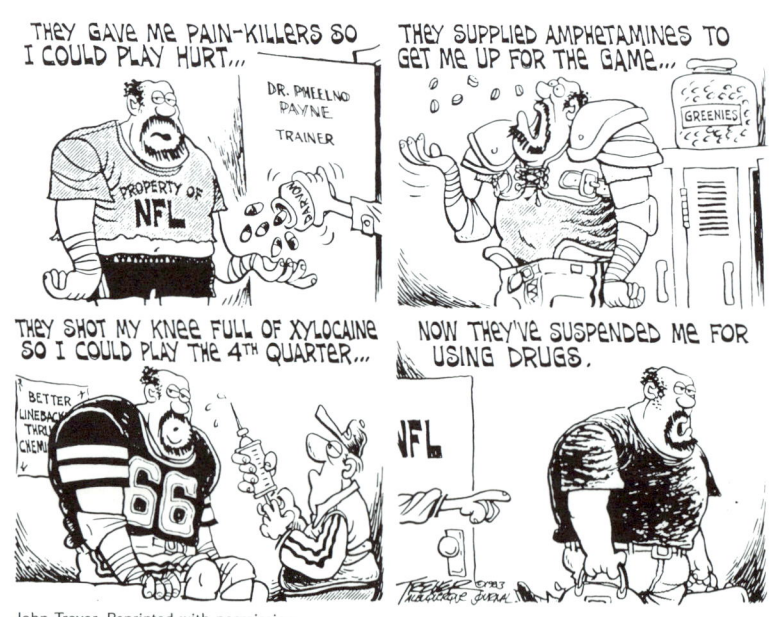

John Trever. Reprinted with permission.

vault higher than bamboo poles. But sports officials did not ban fiberglass poles. Instead, they made the poles available to everyone.

    I, personally, do not believe athletes should take performance-enhancing drugs. As a doctor, I would not prescribe these drugs. But this is my personal opinion, and personal opinion should not decide national policy. Until someone comes up with a good, logical reason for banning performance-enhancing drugs in sports, they should be allowed.

Is inequality among athletes fair?

Some people seem to be born with more athletic ability than others. Do you think it is fair to have athletes with similar abilities compete against each other? Or, do you think it is more fair that everyone gets a chance to compete against all types of athletes? Why?

    Describe a sports situation in which you think one player would have an unfair advantage over another.

VIEWPOINT 4 **Drugs should not be allowed in sports**

Editor's Note: This viewpoint is paraphrased from an article by Thomas H. Murray. Mr. Murray is a professor at the University of Texas. In this viewpoint, Mr. Murray argues against the use of performance-enhancing drugs in sports. He says that athletes are often forced into using drugs even though they are harmful.

Which sentence best expresses the author's main idea in this paragraph?

Usually, when we think of drug users, we think of the spaced-out marijuana smoker. Or we think of the wino sprawled on the curb, or the heroin addict asleep in a doorway. We probably never think of the Olympic gold medalist or the National Football League lineman. Yet these athletes and hundreds of others use performance-enhancing drugs to make them better athletes.

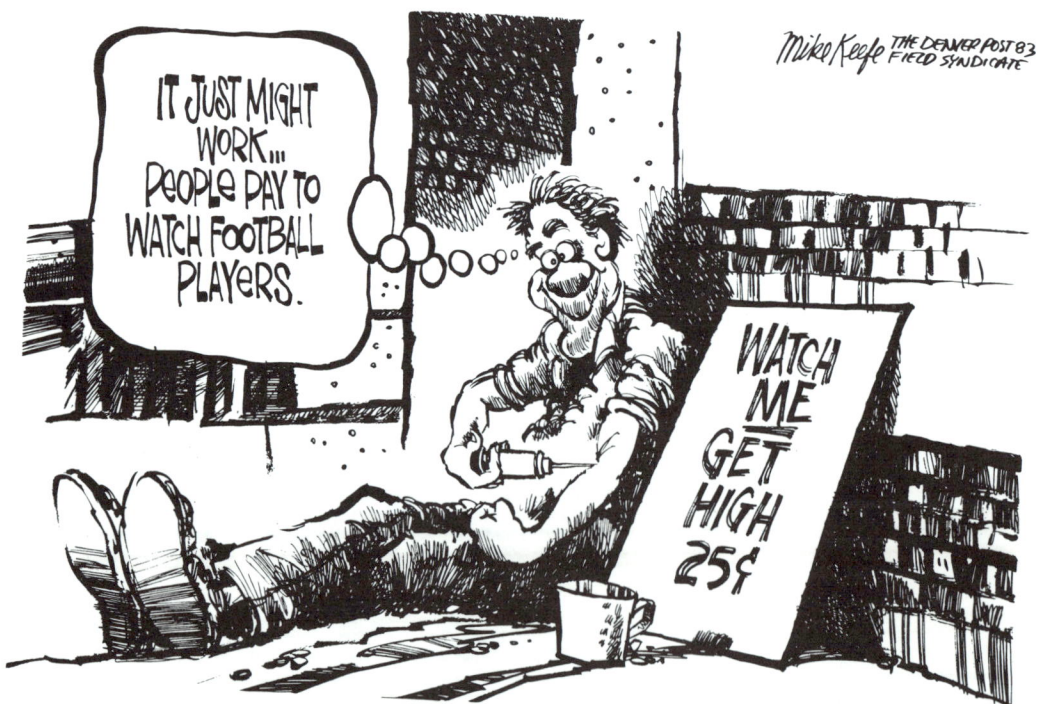

Mike Keefe. Reprinted with permission.

22 JUNIORS

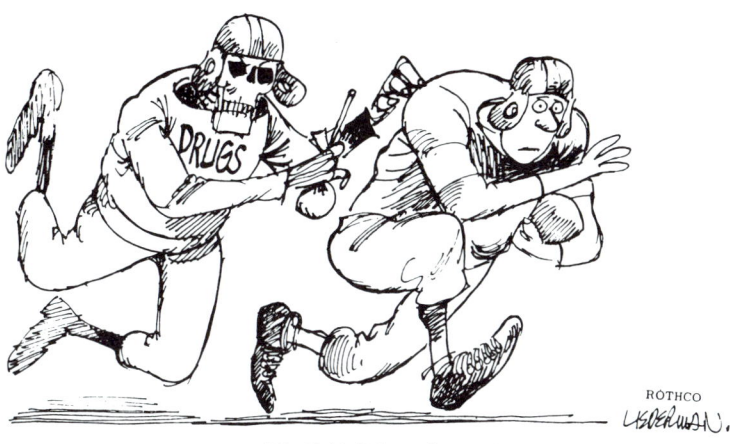

PLAYS FOR KEEPS
© Liederman/Rothco

The use of performance-enhancing drugs should not be allowed in sports. These drugs endanger the athletes' health. They can make them sick both mentally and physically. The International Olympic Committee agrees. The committee prohibits athletes from taking any kind of performance-enhancing drug.

Many athletes take performance-enhancing drugs because they feel they have to take them to compete against other athletes. Sometimes winning is a matter of running to the finish line a fraction of a second before other runners. Sometimes it is a matter of jumping a fraction of an inch farther than other jumpers. When athletes find a drug that gives them an advantage over other athletes, they often give in to the temptation to use it. They want to win, and they will do whatever it takes to win. This includes endangering their health.

Some people say that athletes should be allowed to take drugs if they want to. These people argue that taking drugs is a matter of personal freedom. Athletes and everyone else should be free to do whatever they want with their own bodies.

But what about the freedom of the athletes who do not want to take drugs but feel they must in order to compete? Many athletes spend years training to compete in a sport. Then, when they finally get to the event, they find other athletes are taking performance-enhancing drugs. They know their chances of winning without drugs are slim. They feel forced to take the drugs. This is a serious threat to two of their freedoms—their freedom to remain drug free and their freedom to pursue their life's dreams.

The author's main idea is stated in the first sentence. Do all the remaining sentences in the paragraph support this main idea? Why or why not?

This paragraph contains many ideas. Which sentence best expresses the main point the author is trying to make?

Which sentence best expresses the author's main idea in this paragraph? Do the remaining sentences offer additional information about this main idea? Why or why not?

It is true that there are natural differences between athletes that make them unequal. Ability, dedication, strength, and size all help an athlete to win. But some methods of gaining advantage are unfair. For example, it would be unfair for one runner to take a ten-yard head start. It would also be unfair for one team to have an extra player. It is just as unfair for one athlete to take a performance-enhancing drug when his opponents are competing drug free.

Many people think performance-enhancing drugs are acceptable in sports. Perhaps one reason they tolerate these drugs is that they are so common in our society. Caffeine, for example, is found in coffee, tea, and colas. It is probably the most common drug used by athletes. Caffeine is a stimulant. It perks us up and helps us stay alert. It does the same thing for athletes.

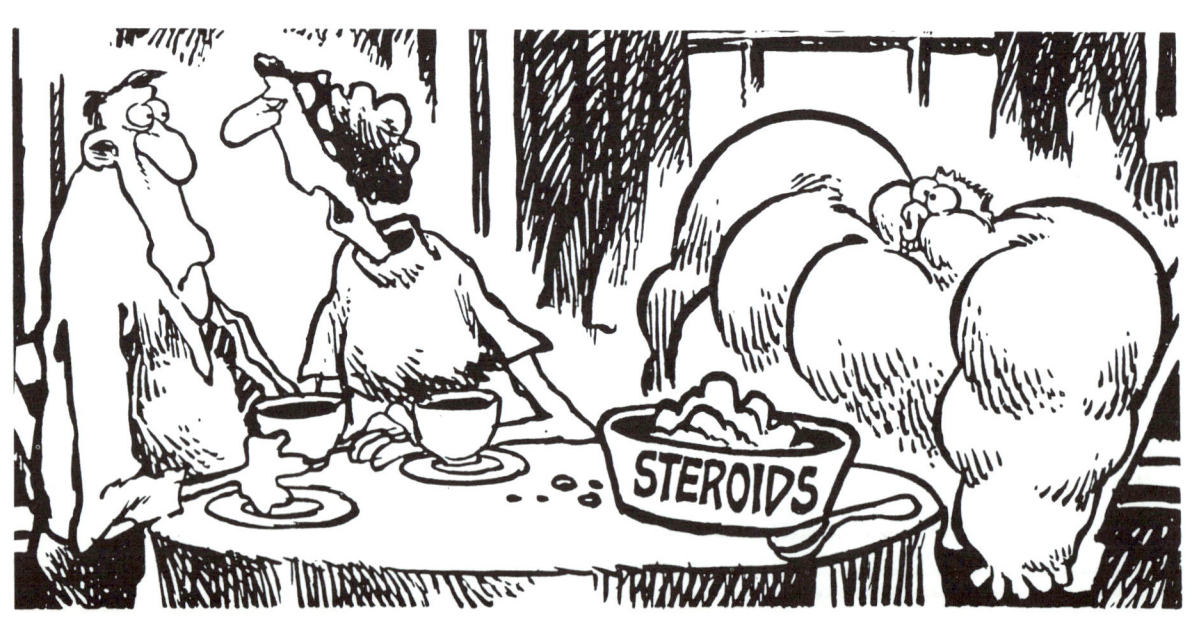

Mike Peters. Reprinted by permission of UFS, Inc.

Maybe taking certain performance-enhancing drugs should be allowed—perhaps even encouraged. But only those drugs that in some way benefit humanity are acceptable. For example, if we had a drug that steadied a surgeon's hand so he or she could operate more safely on a patient, I would favor that drug. If, on the other hand, the drug only allowed the surgeon to operate more quickly and spend more time on the golf course, I would not favor it.

Steroids and other such drugs used by athletes do not benefit everyone. Therefore, these drugs should not be allowed in sports.

> **The main idea of this entire viewpoint is that drugs should not be allowed in sports. Does this paragraph support this main idea? Why or why not?**

> **Do drugs belong in sports?**
>
> Consider the information you have read in viewpoints 3 and 4. Do you think performance-enhancing drugs should be allowed in sports? Why or why not?

CRITICAL THINKING SKILL 2
Identifying the Main Idea in Editorial Cartoons

Throughout this book, you have seen cartoons that illustrate the ideas in the viewpoints. Editorial cartoons are an effective and usually humorous way of presenting an opinion on an issue. Cartoonists sometimes express their main ideas directly. Sometimes, they let the reader determine the main idea of the cartoon by observing clues given in the words and illustration.

Look at the cartoon below. Why has the team's manager recruited a cheerleader, a tuba player, a police officer and a hot dog seller to stand in for the regular football players? What has happened to the regular team members? What is the main idea of this cartoon?

For further practice, look at the editorial cartoons in your daily newspaper. Decide if the cartoonist has stated or implied his or her main idea in the cartoon.

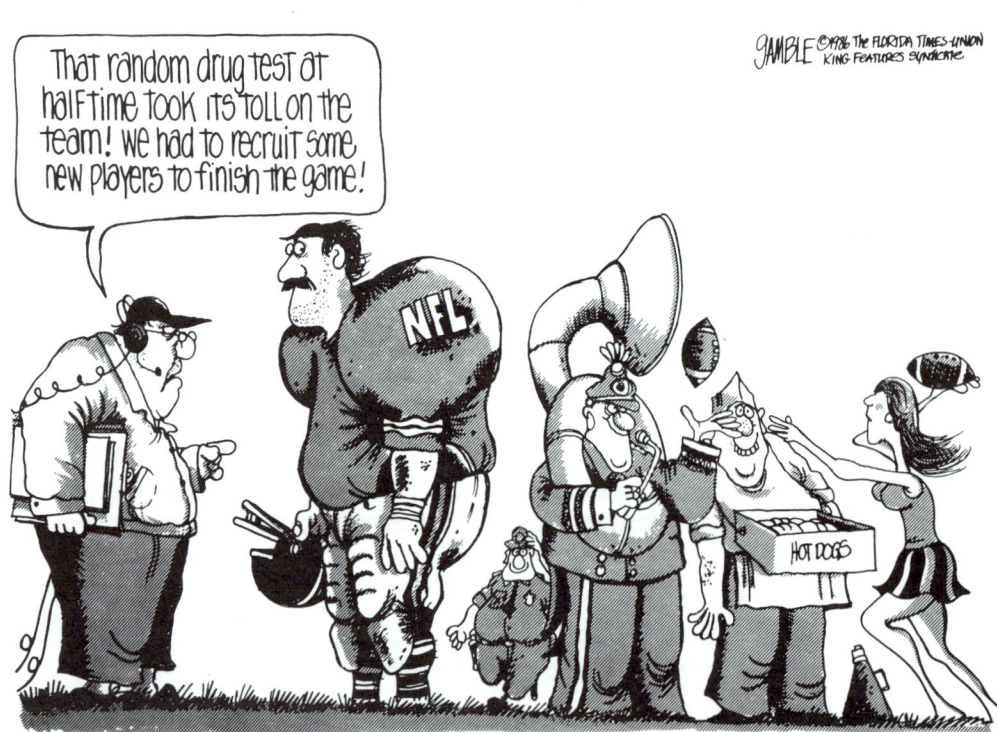

Ed Gamble. Reprinted with permission.

CHAPTER 3

PREFACE: Should Athletes Be Tested for Drug Use?

Many athletes use drugs. They use recreational drugs, such as marijuana and cocaine, to escape the pressures and demands of competitive sports. They use performance-enhancing drugs, such as steroids, to make them stronger. Both types of drugs are dangerous to an athlete's health. To discourage the use of such drugs, many colleges and professional teams have begun testing their players for drugs. Players who test positive for drugs are often suspended and sometimes expelled from their teams.

Some people argue that testing athletes for drugs is necessary. They believe the drug problem in sports has become serious and that something should be done about it. Testing athletes for drugs, they say, would put an end to the problem. It would allow drug experts to come face to face with athletes and educate them about the dangers of using drugs.

Opponents of drug testing believe athletes should not be tested for drugs. They say that the results of these tests are often incorrect. Even if the mistakes are corrected, the athlete's reputation suffers. The public still believes the athlete has a drug problem. People who oppose drug testing say that even if athletes are guilty of using drugs, they should not have to pay for their mistakes forever. But the public never forgives an athlete that has tested positive for drugs. They always remember.

The following viewpoints debate this issue. Read them carefully and locate the author's main ideas in the specified paragraphs.

VIEWPOINT 5 Athletes should be tested for drugs

Editor's Note: This viewpoint is paraphrased from a speech given by Robert Voy, chief medical officer and director of sports medicine and science for the U.S. Olympic Committee. In this speech, Dr. Voy discusses why he believes drug testing is necessary in the world of athletics.

Which sentence best expresses the author's main idea in this paragraph?

No one sentence seems to state the author's main idea. What point is he trying to make in this paragraph?

Athletes should be tested for performance-enhancing drugs. One reason is that it is not fair when some athletes are taking these drugs but others are not. The athletes taking the drugs have an advantage.

But there is an even more important reason for testing athletes for drugs. Athletes will do anything to win, including ruin their health. It is our responsibility to be sure young athletes have an opportunity to participate in sports without damaging their bodies.

One weight lifter had trained for two years to compete in the 1984 Olympics. He took steroids to make him stronger. During the event, he dislocated his elbow. But this was not the worst part. Because steroids strengthen muscles but not tendons, the tendon that controls the lower leg ruptured. The athlete lost control of the weight and the bar hit him in the head. He suffered major injury to his head, leg, and elbow.

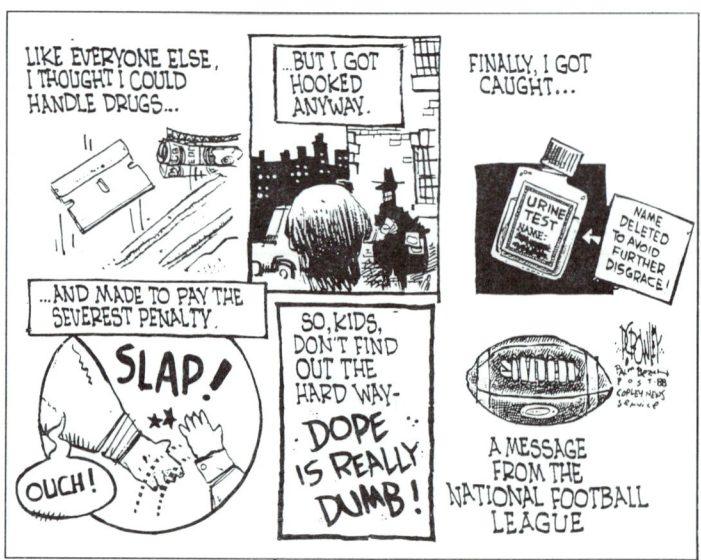

Pat Crowley. Reprinted with permission of Copley News Service.

Athletes must also be protected from other drugs that can poison and even kill them. Our athletes travel all over the world and have access to all sorts of dangerous drugs. Strychnine is a powerful stimulant when used in small amounts. But in large amounts, it is highly poisonous. Strychnine is readily available in South American countries.

Caffeine, available all over the world, is another popular stimulant. Athletes and non-athletes alike use caffeine to boost their energy. But many people do not know that caffeine, when used in large amounts, can be poisonous.

It is true that drugs do enhance performance. Lying to athletes and telling them they do not will not stop them from using them. And athletes will do anything to perform better, even if it means risking their health.

We must do something to save athletes from risking their lives and their health. Do not misunderstand me. We are not going to stop drug abuse in sports or in society just by testing for drugs. But by testing athletes, we come face to face with them. We can teach them something about what they are doing to their bodies. But we cannot do this if we cannot sit down with them and share our knowledge of the harm drugs do to the human body.

What is the author's main idea in this paragraph? Which sentences support the author's main idea?

Does the main idea in this paragraph support the main idea of the whole viewpoint? Why or why not?

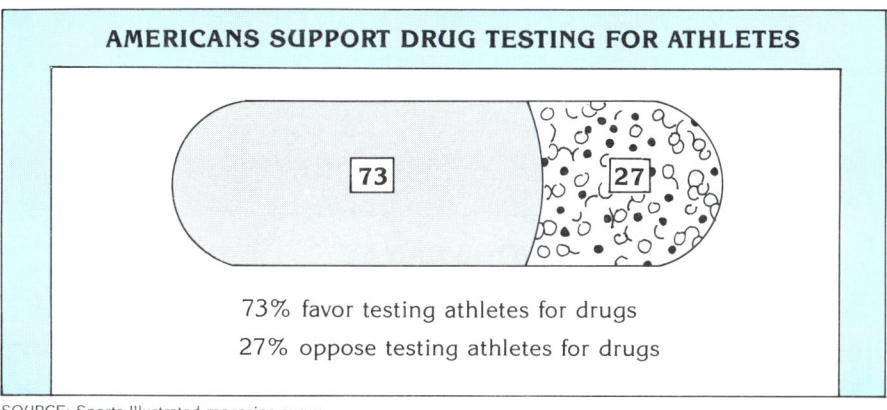

AMERICANS SUPPORT DRUG TESTING FOR ATHLETES

73% favor testing athletes for drugs
27% oppose testing athletes for drugs

SOURCE: Sports Illustrated magazine survey

Would education prevent drug use?

Do you agree with the author that more education would stop athletes from using drugs? Why or why not?

VIEWPOINT 6 **Athletes should not be tested for drugs**

> **Editor's Note:** This viewpoint is paraphrased from an article by Bryan Burwell, a writer for the New York *Daily News*. In it, Mr. Burwell expresses his opinion that drug testing for athletes is unfair.

Which sentences in this paragraph give additional information about the author's main idea?

Does the author's main idea in this paragraph support the main idea of the viewpoint? Why or why not?

The current method of testing athletes for drugs is unfair to the athletes. One reason is that the test results are often incorrect. In one case, traces of the prescription drug codeine, often found in cough syrup, showed up in the systems of several athletes. But someone marked "CO," the symbol for cocaine, on their charts. So several players were labeled cocaine users.

These drug tests are supposed to be kept secret, but team managers and other players sometimes start rumors that some people tested positive. Newspapers find out the names of these people. They print these names, and then the whole country knows about it. This is another reason drug testing is unfair to athletes.

Several athletes have had their reputations ruined when no one has ever proved that they actually did test positive. One example is James FitzPatrick. FitzPatrick was chosen to play for the San Diego Chargers. Two days later, someone spread the rumor that FitzPatrick had tested positive for drugs. Within a day, the story was national news. Now people think he is a drug addict.

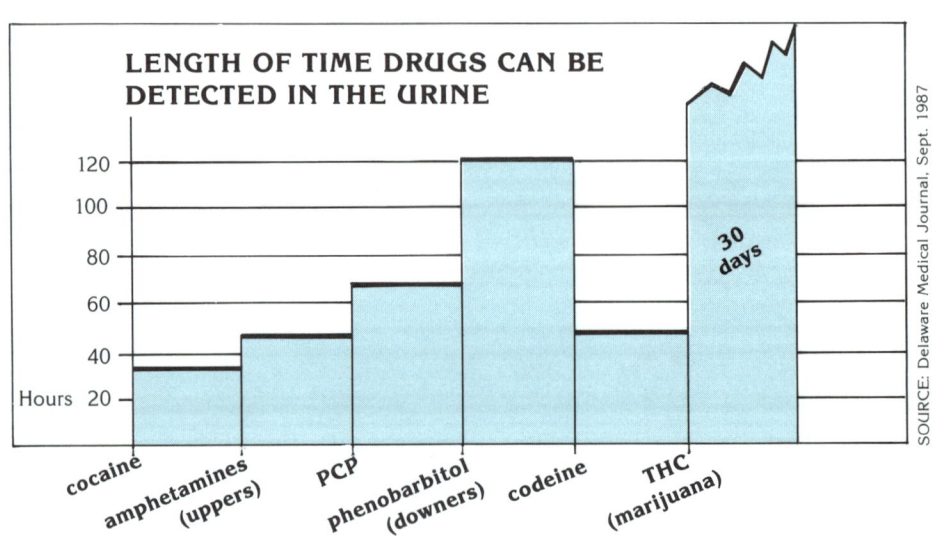

30 JUNIORS

Players lose more than their reputations when people suspect they use drugs. They lose money. Alonzo Johnson, a player for the Philadelphia Eagles, lost about 500 thousand dollars in salary and bonuses because he tested positive for drugs. And players also lose money they might have earned through commercial endorsements. What company would pay an athlete suspected of using drugs to advertise its product?

Even if athletes do test positive for drugs, it is unfair to label them drug addicts for the rest of their lives. Everyone makes mistakes. People should not have to pay for their mistakes forever.

Here is one athlete's story. A football player who did not want to give his name, tested positive for drugs during the National Football League drug tests. Someone in the NFL told the newspapers that he tested positive. So now people call him a drug user.

"Look, I'm not saying what I did was right, because it wasn't," said the athlete. "I smoked some grass. I gave in. I was real depressed at the time. I was wrong. I shouldn't have done it, and now I'm paying for it. But this was supposed to be a private matter—between me and the team, that's all. Now everyone thinks I'm a drug addict and I'm not. But I don't think anyone will ever believe the truth."

The only way drug tests would become fair is if they were done in a special drug-testing facility where the results were kept secret. This change would help future athletes. But it would not help those athletes who have suffered under current testing procedures.

Gene Upshaw, executive director of the NFL Player's Association, put it this way: "The real tragedy is that none of that will help any of these players. Their reputations have already been ruined. It's not fair."

Locate the author's main idea in this paragraph. Do the remaining sentences support the main idea? Why or why not?

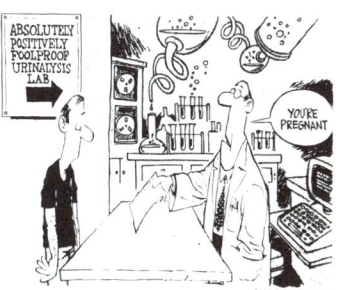

Bob Englehart. Reprinted with permission.

Which sentence best expresses the author's main idea in this paragraph?

Should athletes be tested for drugs?

Do you believe athletes should be tested for drugs? Why or why not?

What two things does the author say athletes lose when the whole country finds out they tested positive for drugs? What is your opinion about athletes who test positive for drugs?

DRUGS AND SPORTS **31**

CRITICAL THINKING SKILL 3

Developing the Main Idea

Below are six main topic ideas. Each is related to the information you have read in these viewpoints. Choose one as a main idea and write a paragraph about it.

EXAMPLE: Topic idea: Athletes sometimes lose money when they take drugs.

Athletes sometimes lose money when they take drugs. Many companies hire athletes to endorse their products. But these companies do not want to hire an athlete whose name is associated with drug use. Also, many athletes who takes drugs are suspended from their teams. They sometimes have to pay fines for taking drugs, and they usually do not get paid while they are on suspension.

Main Ideas:

1. Steroid use is harmful to a person's health.
2. People have the right to use steroids if they want to.
3. If I were an athlete, I would use steroids.
4. If I were an athlete, I would not use steroids.
5. Drugs should not be allowed in sports.
6. Athletes should be tested for drugs.